THE BEGINNERS' BOOK OF ESSENTIAL OILS

LEARNING TO USE YOUR FIRST 10 ESSENTIAL OILS WITH CONFIDENCE

A BEGINNER'S GUIDE TO ESSENTIAL OILS WITH 80+ RECIPES TO GET YOU STARTED

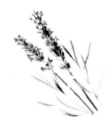

©2015, Christine Dalziel

Joybilee Farm Media

British Columbia, Canada

ISBN Print version
13:978-1511977180
10:1511977183

DISCLAIMER: *This book is for educational purposes only. I am not a doctor, a nurse, nor a nutritionist. While I have spent many years learning about herbs and essential oils, and researching their properties, I am not a clinical herbalist. This book is not intended to diagnose, treat, nor prescribe. Statements made in this book have not been approved by any government agency.*

While herbs and essential oils are not drugs, they need to be treated with respect as to their potency and appropriateness to pregnant and nursing mothers and young children. Please consult your personal physician or naturopath for your personal and family health needs. I am not responsible for any claims, damages, losses, judgements, expenses, costs, injuries, actions, or outcome resulting from the use of the information or recipes in this book.

Dedication:

This book is dedicated to Robin, Christopher, Ian, and Sarah. You walked with me through more than 30 years of education, through trial and error, through research, and through practical experience, learning how to best use these essential oils for vibrant health, for the well-being of our livestock and pets, and for our own healing journey. These essential oils are an integral part of who we are, our family memories, and our efforts mip'nei tikkun ha-olam (תקון עולם). Remember how well tea tree oil and lavender helped with those nasty wasp stings? Remember the sweet smell of peppermint and eucalyptus in the bathtub when you were sick? Remember the sleepytime spritz of lavender on your pillow at bedtime, to chase away the stress and bad dreams? I hope as you remember you also remember how much I love you. I hope you enjoy this humble gift intended to bless you and fill you with JOY and happy memories.

"The way to health is to have an aromatic bath and a scented massage every day," advised Hippocrates around 400 BC. If the father of modern medicine was correct, most of us would be doomed to weakness and disease. Who has time for an aromatic bath? Who can afford a daily massage? And they charge more if you want essential oils added. Hippocrates was pointing to the value of aromatic plants in health and wellbeing. A modern corollary would be "eat more flowers."

The use of aromatic plants is the oldest form of medicine. Oil, alcohol, honey, and vinegar infused with fragrant plants were used in every culture for health, beauty, and cleansing, as well as for spiritual practice. These infused products became the basis for salves, ointments, medicine, and healing balms in herbal medicinal traditions, as well as fragrant perfumes and incense. But these are not essential oils. Essential oils are the product of steam distillation, rather than infusion.

Steam distillation of essential oils from aromatic plants is a fairly recent invention. Developed by the Ottoman Turks, it was a well-guarded secret, until their monopoly was broken in WW I. This is the same time that scientific inquiry was entering a new era and separating itself from the work of the alchemist. This was when the intellectual and scientific demarcations in various schools of knowledge were hardened.

While there is a long tradition of using aromatic plants for medicine that spans thousands of years, the use of essential oils is just a few hundred years old. Further, scientific inquiry and double blind studies in the efficacy of essential oils are less than 100 years old. While this may seem inadequate, one must understand that all scientific inquiry with the double blind experimental standard is just over 100 years old. My husband's Great Uncle, Dr. Alexander Crum Brown (1838 - 1922), was one of the first organic chemists in the world, at a time when "science" just meant knowledge. His great contribution was the insistence that mathematics must be an integral part of chemistry and scientific discovery.

Put in that perspective, we understand that our current scientific dogmas are relatively new. While many point to evidence based scientific inquiry as the standard that every herb or aromatic plant must adhere to before it can be used for health, plants have had a symbiotic relationship with mankind for millennium. There is value in the scientific method and there is also value in tradition and personal experience. It is not one to the exclusion of the other. It isn't that way in any other branch of knowledge, not even in allopathic medicine. It's important that we don't put a burden of proof on traditional medicine that we don't put on allopathic medicine. The gold standard of double blind studies is useful, but only part of the bigger picture.

I encourage you, as you begin to explore the value of essential oils, that you keep notes of both evidence based information, as well as traditional and personal experience in your study of herbs. In this way you will gain the full picture of what herbs and essential oils have to offer you and your family. You will mature in your understanding of when to use essential oils, when to choose a different herbal preparation, and when to seek professional advice.

My personal interest in essential oils began over 30 years ago, when I created my first batch of soap using lavender essential oil. In those years, before the internet, essential oils came in 5ml bottles displayed at the checkout of my local health food store. If I wanted to buy essential oils in larger quantities, I had to special order them. There were no standards and the Latin name wasn't on the bottle. Lavender was lavender. Eucalyptus was eucalyptus. We had no way of deciding which variety of eucalyptus we were getting. And we didn't know it mattered.

When my vaccinated 2 year old came down with whooping cough in the middle of the night, we ran hot water in the claw foot iron bath tub to create lots of steam and shook droplets of eucalyptus, rosemary, and marjoram essential oils into the tub to loosen her phlegm and let her breathe. No one advised this treatment. We weren't cautioned against certain varieties of eucalyptus being dangerous for young children. Desperate moms do things out of instinct, or because their own mom did that, not from reading scientific journals. Surprisingly, that little 2 year old grew up to be a beautiful young woman. Her illness was short. We had a couple of scary nights and she fully recovered in just a few days.

During the time that I wrote this book, I visited a Chinese smorgasbord and got a tiny piece of almond, from the almond chicken, caught under my tooth, below the gum. It was mildly irritating. We were away from home and it was several hours before I was able to get it out using dental floss. It was uncomfortable at the time but manageable. That was on a Wednesday night. Saturday morning my mouth was a little sore, but I attributed it to not sleeping well. By Sunday it turned into a painful infection. On Monday I woke up to an abscessed tooth. That was so painful that just grazing the top molar with my tongue sent shooting pains into my brain.

Although I ignored the minor irritation at first, once it was abscessed it had my full attention. I applied clove essential oil to numb the pain and tea tree essential oil to deal with the infection. The essential oils relieved the nerve pain and pressure overnight, though it didn't make it vanish. A dull ache remained and I couldn't chew. Over the next few days, with the help of some herbal tinctures, colloidal silver, oil pulling, and continued applications of tea tree and myrrh essential oils, the toothache subsided. I didn't need to visit a dentist, though I would have if the herbal remedies didn't take care of the problem so quickly.

The purpose of this short book is to help you find that path from knowledge to instinct. I want you to have confidence in your use of essential oils, so that when a problem arises that essential oils can help with, you know which ones to choose and how to apply them. While scientific studies are valuable, most are out of reach on closely guarded science websites that only the elite have access to. But even doctors, armed with access to the latest research, still rely on personal experience (and drug company reps) to guide them in their practice of medicine.

And so we mothers must learn to rely on our own wisdom and experience to guide our decisions, even more so, as bureaucrats, rather than doctors are making medical decisions for our families.

My hope is that this book will guide you in your growing exploration of essential oils, so that you can add to your experience with them, and get to know them intimately. While they are not the last word on effective herbal remedies, my hope is that you will incorporate them into your daily life and practice, and that they won't become a last resort. Essential oils are an important part of holistic health techniques and I hope this book gives you the confidence to use them well.

CONTENTS

I'm often asked which essential oils should someone who is new to using essential oils start with. I recommend these 10 oils most often because they are nontoxic, easy to use, generally considered safe, and adapted to many uses.

- Lavender
- Lemon
- Peppermint
- Tea Tree
- Rosemary
- Eucalyptus
- Marjoram
- Rose Geranium
- Frankincense
- Myrrh

These 10 essential oils span the full range of scents from sweetly floral, to bright menthol, and pungent balsam. They give cheering top notes, balancing middle notes, and long lasting base notes to fragrant or therapeutic blends. They offer a full range of beneficial actions to strengthen the immune system and hasten healing, relief, and comfort.

Another advantage of these 10 beginner essential oils is that they are generally safe for external use. They can be used by pregnant and nursing mothers, and with just a few exceptions, which I mention, can be used for children and babies.

ODOR PRINT

Have you ever noticed that when you visit people there is a lingering scent that you begin to associate with them and their house? This is called an "odor print." In many homes it comes from chemical laundry detergent and fabric softener, and permeates their carpets and living space with toxic fumes. Forget those toxic solid room fresheners that only mask repulsive odors. When you use essential oils you control the odor print of your home. Instead of toxic chemicals you can choose natural scents for their calming, centering, or energizing qualities.

Further, essential oils actually cleanse room air of toxins, bacteria, and viruses. They do this in the same way that a salt lamp or a beeswax candle does. They release negative ions into the air. Since bacteria, viruses, and petroleum-based chemicals have positive ions, these are neutralized by essential oils. Essential oils leave your home smelling healthy.

If you work in an environment where you are exposed to bacteria, viruses, and molds and are prone to become sick with whatever is going around, diffusing essential oils at home, may be the edge you need. Teachers, nurses, medics, civil servants, pastors, rabbis, and students benefit from essential oils diffused in their homes.

Begin with just a few essential oils and learn them well. Use them for air fresheners, put them in your essential oil diffuser, add them to skin care products, cosmetics, tooth powders, mouthwash, and home cleaning products. Pay attention to how you feel when you smell them. Are they calming? Do they help you sleep? Do they make you more focused and alert? While essential oils have a specific effect on most people, not everyone reacts the same way. If you loath the scent of lavender, you may be one of the people that don't react the usual way with it. Other calming and balancing oils, like geranium essential oil can replace lavender.

If you were going to start with only 3 essential oils, I'd suggest lavender, lemon, and peppermint. Lavender contributes calm, antibacterial, antifungal, and skin healing effects. Lemon adds its antibacterial, antimicrobial, anti-depressant effects. Peppermint offers its bright, energizing, antibacterial, and uplifting character.

Then if I was going to add three more to these three, I'd add tea tree, rosemary, and eucalyptus. Tea Tree has antimicrobial and bug repelling actions. Rosemary increases alertness and memory. Eucalyptus helps during a cold, to loosen congestion and free breathing, as well as being antimicrobial. If I had young children I'd choose **Eucalyptus radiata** , over other varieties because it is considered safer for very young children. Keep in mind that moms have been using Eucalyptus to help their babies breathe more freely for generations; even when essential oils came in 5ml bottles at the apothecary. These 6 essential oils are the ones I go to over and over again for scent, for cleaning, for first aid, and for skin care.

The other four essential oils, marjoram, geranium, frankincense, and myrrh, I'd add on an as needed basis. As you have a recipe that uses them, purchase them for your essential oils kit. You can create a lot of recipes with essential oils using just the first 6.

A WORD ABOUT CITRUS ESSENTIAL OILS

Citrus oils are cold pressed from the peels of oranges, lemons, and other citrus fruit. All citrus essential oils have similar actions. They are all bright, cheering scents. They all have antimicrobial and astringent benefits. But their scents are short lived. They won't linger in your home in the same way that lavender or peppermint does. If you aren't partial to lemon, pick the citrus scent that most appeals to you. There are a lot of choices in citrus scents. You can also choose two or more citrus oils and combine them according to your preference. If a recipe calls for 12 drops of lemon essential oil, you can create your own blend by substituting 4 drops each of grapefruit, sweet orange, and lemon, for instance. Do what pleases your own nose and sense of balance. The fugitive nature of citrus essential oils can be stabilized in a blend by using a fixative like myrrh essential oil.

While it might be nice to have 100 different essential oils in a pretty carrying case, having 10 essential oils that you know confidentially is more beneficial than having 100 oils that you never use. Start small. Learn your oils intimately by using them. Add more essential oils as you need them. Don't be attracted by the bling. Save your money. Invest in just these 10 and build a strong foundation of essential oil knowledge and practical experience before you branch out.

HOW TO STORE YOUR ESSENTIAL OILS

Essential oils are considered essential because they are volatile in the air. They evaporate easily when they are exposed to air. In your body, they break down quickly, enter your blood stream, are removed by your liver and excreted. While they enter your blood stream within minutes, in 2 hours from the time you first smell them, they are on their way out. This makes them fast acting and prevents toxicity in your body, which is healthy for you. They do present some challenges, however, for adequate storage.

When you store essential oils in your house, they can break down quickly, if they aren't stored properly. Each time you open the bottle, you lose a little bit into the air. If you buy them in large bottles, some of the precious oil is wasted each time you open the bottle. So transfer your oils to smaller, nonreactive amber or blue glass bottles and use a drop reducer lid to protect the oils. This will protect your investment.

If your oils come with a dropper, remove the dropper from the bottle for storage and replace it with a drop reducer and an airtight cap. Some essential oils will eat through the flexible rubber top of a dropper, ruining your oil.

Make small amounts of each essential oil recipe. You may be tempted to double or triple the batch, but the volatile essential oils will evaporate from the product as it is exposed to air. Smaller jars and bottles are better than large jars and bottles for storage.

Don't store your essential oils or the products that you make in plastic, if you have a choice. Many of the essential oils will break down plastic. Instead save small jars from jam or honey and reuse these to store your homemade essential oil products. My maple syrup comes in tall 1 quart glass bottles. When I make my spray cleaners I use these glass bottles and replace the lid with a spray cap. It makes my cleaner last just a little longer in the bottle.

You may find that the reducer cap on your essential oils bottles becomes hardened and clogged by resinous essential oils like myrrh or frankincense. Tea Tree can dissolve the soft plastic of a reducer cap, as well. As this becomes problematic replace the reducer cap with a fresh one. This will extend the life of your essential oils.

Used but sound essential oil bottles, reducer caps, and lids can be washed in hot soapy water and reused. The essential oils can be rinsed out and the bottles air dried. Use these recycled essential oil bottles to store perfume blends and diffuser blends.

HOW LONG WILL MY ESSENTIAL OILS LAST?

While large bottles in the 500 ml range may seem like a bargain, don't purchase essential oils in larger quantities than you can use in a year or two. Essential oils have a shelf life, just like all plant based substances. After a year you may notice the smell of an essential oil degrading. If it still smells strong and fresh, you may continue using it. However, if you notice the smell degrading, **use it for cleaning products** rather than putting it on your body and purchase fresh essential oil for your beauty and health products. You don't need to toss it, just change how you plan to use it up.

Citrus essential oils seem to oxidize sooner than other essential oils. They are more volatile in the air. Buy them in the amounts that you can use up in a year. You can extend the shelf life of citrus oils by keeping them refrigerated. Storing at cooler temperatures does prolong their shelf life and delay oxidization.

Some essential oils are diluted in a carrier oil when you purchase them. Blended essential oils and the more expensive absolutes are often blended with carrier oils to reduce the cost. The carrier oil can become rancid in these bottles. If the scent of the essential oil becomes off or rancid, use it for cleaning products only or discard it. Don't put rancid oil on your skin and don't ingest it. Rancid oils are harmful to you and your family.

HOW TO DISCARD EXPIRED OR RANCID ESSENTIAL OILS

There is no away. Everything you bring into your home eventually needs to be responsibly discarded. This includes drugs, cleaning supplies, herbs, and essential oils. This job becomes easier when you make a point of only purchasing **certified organic essential oils**. Organic essential oils will be processed without harsh solvents, usually through steam distillation or cold pressing. Organic essential oils however, are a concentrated and highly antimicrobial substance. They need special treatment when you dispose of them.

Don't dump expired essential oils down the drain or into your septic tank. The volatile oils can cause problems in the microbial rich environment of a septic system. To safely discard certified organic essential oils, pour them over sawdust or wood chips and scatter them in the pathways of your garden. They will safely enter the environment without causing damage to the eco system. Do not put them in a compost pile, a worm bin, nor flush them down the drain. These environments are not suitable for the strong antimicrobial action of many essential oils. Since the oils break down quickly in the environment, you'll notice that the strong scent dissipates rapidly once it is exposed to air.

By planning ahead and only purchasing the essential oils that you can reasonably use within the expiry period you will have less need to dispose of them. Throwing essential oils on the ground is like tossing your money in the garbage. Plan wisely.

CARRIER OILS

Essential oils are concentrated plant chemicals. A single drop represents many pounds of plant material focused at a single point.

In all but a very few circumstances essential oils should be diluted with a carrier oil before being applied to your skin. This prevents sensitization as well as slowing down the absorption of the essential oil.

Use organic carrier oils without a strong scent of their own. Sweet almond oil, grapeseed oil, hazelnut oil, and coconut oil are all good choices. While it has a scent of its own, I also often use virgin olive oil. Your body will absorb the carrier oil along with the essential oil, so avoid using oils that you wouldn't ingest or that you have an allergy to. The following chart gives standard dilutions for essential oils. Note that 1 drop of essential oil in 1 tsp. of carrier oil is a 1% dilution.

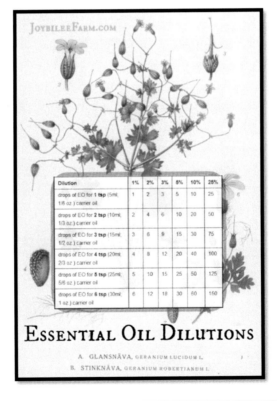

JOYBILEEFARM.COM

Dilution	1%	2%	3%	5%	10%	25%
drops of EO for **1 tsp** (5ml, 1/6 oz.) carrier oil	1	2	3	5	10	25
drops of EO for **2 tsp** (10ml, 1/3 oz.) carrier oil	2	4	6	10	20	50
drops of EO for **3 tsp** (15ml, 1/2 oz.) carrier oil	3	6	9	15	30	75
drops of EO for **4 tsp** (20ml, 2/3 oz.) carrier oil	4	8	12	20	40	100
drops of EO for **5 tsp** (25ml, 5/6 oz.) carrier oil	5	10	15	25	50	125
drops of EO for **6 tsp** (30ml, 1 oz.) carrier oil	6	12	18	30	60	150

ESSENTIAL OIL DILUTIONS

A. GLANSNÄVA, GERANIUM LUCIDUM L.

B. STINKNÄVA, GERANIUM ROBERTIANUM L.

Several recipes in this book call for infused oils. While you can purchase these infused oils from **Mountain Rose Herbs,** you can also make them yourself. To make an infused oil, simply add 1 cup of dried herbs to 2 cups of a suitable carrier oil. Allow it to macerate in a warm place for 4 weeks. Shake the tightly capped jar once a day. After 4 weeks, strain it through a sieve to remove the spent plant material. Put it in a clean jar and label. You can use this infused oil in the place of a carrier oil in any of these recipes. Suitable herbs for infusion include chamomile, calendula or St. John's Wort flowers, and comfrey, plantain, or eucalyptus leaves.

When preparing a remedy for very young children, use your already infused oils or you can infuse carrier oils with plant materials, as needed, to **replace** an essential oil in some preparations. For instance, with chest congestion in infants try infusing eucalyptus leaves and peppermint leaves in a carrier oil, rather than using the essential oils, where the essential oils may have unwanted effects. You can speed the maceration time by heating the oil in a covered crock pot overnight. Keep the temperature below boiling to preserve the volatile plant oils within the carrier oil. Cool the oil and strain it. Bottle it and label it. It can now be used effectively in place of carrier oil and essential oils when you are making a cold remedy for young children, where you don't want to use peppermint or eucalyptus essential oils.

Infused oils are not the same as essential oils. While essential oils are distilled volatile oils from aromatic plant sources, infused oils have a lesser concentration of volatile oils, but also contain oil soluble fractions of the herb, that aren't included in the essential oil. **This is an important distinction.** If you are reading about an herbal medicinal benefit that makes use of a whole plant extract, it is a mistake to infer that the essential oil alone can substitute for the use of the whole herb. The volatile oil is just one part of the whole herb. When using herbs medicinally based on a scientific study it's important to determine which part of the plant was used in the study, before you use herbs in the hope for a cure. This is especially true when evaluating the health claims made by essential oils sales reps.

When you use infused oil or an herbal extraction you gain the benefit of using more of the herb. For instance when making an antimicrobial all-purpose cleaner, many people will put ¼ tsp of clove essential oil, lemon essential oil, rosemary essential oil, and cinnamon essential oil into vinegar for their strong antimicrobial actions. A better all-purpose cleaner can be made by infusing lemon peels, whole cloves, cinnamon sticks, and rosemary branches in vinegar and macerating in a warm place for 4 to 8 weeks. The resulting all-purpose cleaner has more grease cutting, and grime dissolving capability as well as the antimicrobial action of the essential oils alone. Why not use both whole herbs AND essential oils and expand your repertoire of herbal benefits?

While this book is specific to using essential oils, consider adding infused oils, infused vinegars, tinctures, and herbal extracts to your repertoire of DiY beauty, health, and cleaning projects. The ideal herbal would include the use of whole herbs as well as essential oils.

A WORD ABOUT ALLERGIES

Contrary to popular opinion, essential oils can cause allergies and sensitivities even though they don't contain proteins. If you are unsure please test each essential oil before you apply it to your body or your child's body. To test for essential oil sensitivities place 1 drop of essential oil in 1 tsp of carrier oil to make a 1% dilution of the essential oil. Put a very tiny amount of this on the inside of your forearm or the inside of your thigh. Cover it with a bandage and wait 24 hours. If you notice any redness, swelling, or rash develop, proceed very cautiously. You may be sensitive to that essential oil (or the carrier oil). Do not use an essential oil that you are sensitive to, without discussing it with your personal medical practitioner.

LET'S GET TO KNOW YOUR 10 NEW OILS.

You learn best when you engage your eyes, your hands, and your nose, as you explore essential oils. I encourage you to go beyond just following the recipes in this book. Smell, touch, and write down your experiences in the notes. I include places to write down your impressions and experiences with each of these 10 essential oils. Record where you purchased each one, the price that you paid, and whether you found the quality appropriate for your needs. This information will help you make wise decisions in the future.

Also include your personal experience with each oil and with them in combination. If you are a sensitive soul with multiple allergies, please test each essential oil for allergic reactions using a 1% solution on the inside of your forearm. (1 drop of essential oil in 1 tsp. carrier oil) Wait 24 hours and check for allergy or sensitivity before using the essential oil in one of the recipes. If you experience any redness, rash, or other allergic reaction, forgo that particular essential oil and make an annotation in the note section of this book for future guidance.

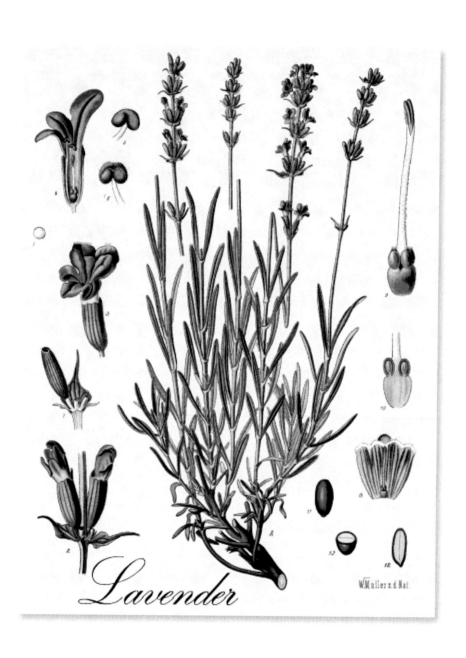

Lavender

W. Müller n.d. Nat.

(Lavandula agustifolia)

Lavender is calming, pain relieving, and anti-spasmodic. It is anti-inflammatory, anti-microbial, antifungal, and antibacterial. Lavender aids digestion and supports the liver. Uniquely, it is both a sedative and a stimulant so it relaxes without making you groggy. It also helps to reduce fever. And it encourages menstruation, when there is blockage. It calms the nerves and emotions and brings them into balance. It is insecticidal and was historically used as a moth repellent. If you have a minor burn or sunburn, apply lavender and the pain will subside, the tissue will repair, often without scarring.

Lavender is one of the few essential oils that can be applied directly on the skin without a carrier oil to dilute it. While those with sensitive skin should use a carrier oil, to prevent sensitization, those with hardier constitutions can get away with applying it neat to the skin. I keep a small vial of lavender essential oil, with a roller ball to apply to wounds, insect stings, and burns. A bee sting can be rendered painless and the swelling reduced with the immediate application of lavender essential oil.

LAVENDER

- Analgesic

- Antibacterial

- Anti-depressant

- Anti-emetic
- Antifungal
- Anti-inflammatory
- Anti-microbial
- Antiseptic
- Anti-spasmodic
- Aromatic
- Carminative
- Cholagogue
- Deodorant
- Digestive
- Diuretic
- Emmenagogue
- Insecticide
- Nervine
- Rubefacient
- Sedative
- Stimulant
- Vulnerary

Lavender provides a **middle note** in blends.

USES FOR LAVENDER ESSENTIAL OIL:

USE IT IN THE LAUNDRY

Add a few drops to your wool dryer balls to make your laundry smell fresh and clean.

IRONING SPRAY

Add 10 drops of lavender essential oil to a spray bottle of filtered water to spray linen tablecloths and pillow cases before ironing. It will make the job of ironing more pleasant and keep your linens smelling fresh and clean.

BURN AND FIRST AID OINTMENT

Use lavender essential oil in a burn ointment for sunburn

> 2 tbsp. of calendula infused oil
> 10 drops of lavender essential oil

Mix together in a 30 ml bottle. Label. Shake well before use. Apply to minor cuts, scrapes, and burns to speed healing, relieve pain, and provide an antimicrobial barrier to prevent infection.

PROMOTES RELAXATION AND SLEEP

Diffuse lavender essential oil in a bedroom to help induce deep sleep and especially to promote REM sleep and encourage dreaming. Lavender relaxes the mind and encourages the healing phase of sleep. It also relaxes brain activity helping to calm the mind and emotions.

HELPS EASE A HEADACHE

A drop of lavender essential oil applied to the temples can ease a tension headache in a few minutes.

SPEEDS WOUND HEALING

Add a drop of lavender to a bandage and place over a cut to disinfect and speed wound healing.

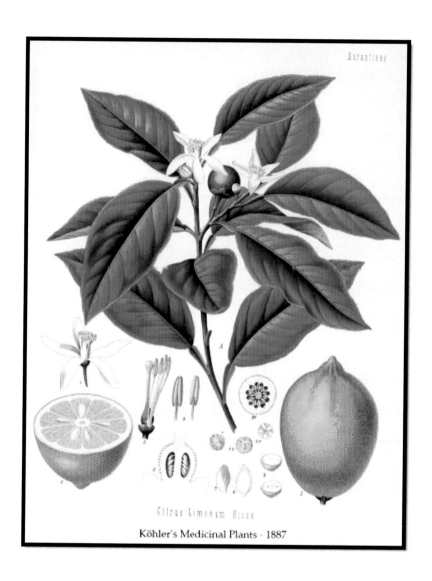

Köhler's Medicinal Plants - 1887

(Citrus limon)

Lemon and the other citrus essential oils like sweet orange, bergamot, lime, and grapefruit can be used interchangeable. Pick the scents that you like best. Bergamot seems longer lasting to me than lemon, grapefruit, or sweet orange. Using a base note like myrrh or frankincense as a fixative can improve the lasting power of citrus scents.

Citrus essential oils are cold pressed from the peels of ripe citrus fruit, unlike other essential oils that are steam distilled. The shelf life of citrus oils can be prolonged by storing the coloured glass bottles in the refrigerator, inhibiting oxidization.

Lemon is antiseptic. It stimulates digestion by supporting the liver. It prevents contagious illnesses like colds and flu when it is diffused into room air. It is refreshing, uplifting, and anti-depressant. I like to use lemon essential oils in my homemade cleaning products for the refreshing scent that it gives my home.

LEMON

- Antibacterial

- Antifungal

- Anti-microbial

- Anti-parasitic

- Antiseptic

- Anti-inflammatory

- Anti-rheumatic

- Anti-spasmodic

- Astringent

- Carminative

- Digestive

- Diuretic

- Insecticidal

- Laxative

- Sedative

- Tonic

- Restorative

USES FOR LEMON ESSENTIAL OIL

Lemon essential oil is a natural degreaser and antimicrobial. It is an excellent addition to all your homemade cleaners. If you prefer another citrus scent like grapefruit or sweet orange, you can substitute one of these for the lemon essential oil called for in the recipes in this book, without loss of effectiveness.

Lemon adds a **top note** to essential oil and perfume blends.

MOSQUITO REPELLANT

Add 10 drops of lemon essential oil to ½ cup of witch hazel. Place in a spritz bottle to repel mosquitos.

WOOD CONDITIONER

Put 12 drops of lemon or other citrus oil in ¼ c.walnut oil and use it to condition wooden spoons, cutting boards, and other wooden kitchen tools. Wipe on, allow it to absorb for 10 to 15 minutes. Wipe excess oil off and buff dry.

AIR CLEANER

Diffuse lemon, grapefruit, or orange essential oil in a room to elevate mood, and clean the air of viruses and bacteria.

DISINFECTANT

Put 4 drops of lemon essential oil on a cloth and wipe door knobs, light switches, and keyboards to disinfect without water.

HAND SOFTENER

Mix together 1 tbsp. of sea salt, 1 tbsp. of coconut oil or sweet almond oil, and 6-8 drops of lemon essential oil. Rub salt-oil mixture on hands, paying attention to calluses and cuticles. Massage in for 1 minute. Rinse in warm water. Pat dry.

HAIRBRUSH AND COMB CONDITIONER

Put 5 drops of lemon essential oil into a sink of hot water. After cleaning combs and brushes of discarded hair and lint, soak combs and brushes for 15 minutes. Rinse and air dry.

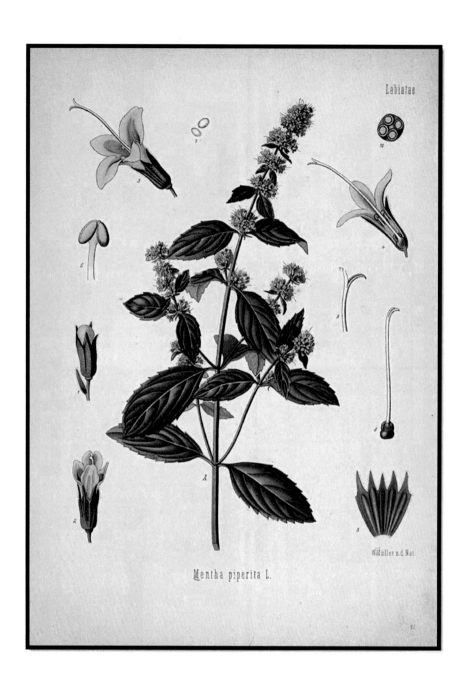

Labiatae

Mentha piperita L.

WMüller n.d. Nat.

(*Mentha piperita*)

Peppermint is bright, bold, and uplifting. It will lift your mood, and energize you while it reduces stress. Peppermint will calm an upset stomach or a headache. It reduces pain. It strengthens. It clears the sinuses and is stimulating. A single drop can alleviate motion sickness. It should be used sparingly in blends for best effect. **It should not be used for children under 3 years old due to its strong menthol content**. For very young children infuse a carrier oil with peppermint leaves and use that oil rather than the much more concentrated essential oil.

PEPPERMINT

- Analgesic

- Anti-parasitic

- Antiseptic

- Astringent

- Carminative

- Cholagogue

- Cordial

- Digestive

- Emmenagogue

- Expectorant

- Febrifuge

- Insecticidal

- Nervine

- Sedative

- Stimulant

- Stomachic

- Vasoconstrictor

Peppermint adds a **top note** to essential oil blends and perfumes.

USES FOR PEPPERMINT ESSENTIAL OIL

BREATH FRESHENER

In a purse size spray bottle mix 1 tbsp. of distilled water and 2 drops of peppermint essential oil.   To use shake well, and spritz the tongue to freshen breathe. It will be strong so use sparingly.

TOOTHPASTE

Mix 1 tbsp. of coconut oil, 1 tbsp. of baking soda, and 3 drops of peppermint essential oil. Mix well. Put in a small jar. Use this to moisten your toothbrush and brush your teeth. It freshens your breath, cleans your teeth, and helps with gum disease.

FOOT MASSAGE OIL

For tired, achy feet, put 1 tsp of coconut oil and 1 drop of peppermint essential oil in your palm. Allow the coconut oil to melt with your body heat. Massage into the bottoms of your feet, to cool, refresh, and ease tension.

STUDYING LATE AT NIGHT

Put 4 to 8 drops of peppermint essential oil into a room diffuser to keep you alert while you are studying into the wee hours of the night. Peppermint will help you stay alert without the caffeine hit and jittery after-effects of adrenal fatigue.

CLAY POULTICE FOR ARTHRITIS RELIEF

When Arthur comes to visit make a clay poultice of 1 tbsp. French green clay and warm water. Add 3 drops of peppermint essential oil, 1 drop of lavender essential oil, and 3 drops of rosemary essential oil. Mix to form a stiff paste. Smear the mixture over the affected joints and painful areas. Cover with muslin and keep warm. Leave on for 20 minutes. Rinse and dry. This draws out the toxins and increases circulation in the joints, bringing relief.

DISCOURAGE MICE AND RATS FROM YOUR HOME

Dissuade mice from making your home into theirs by planting peppermint plants around the perimeter of your home and creating a perfume of 30% peppermint essential oil, 30% alcohol and 40% distilled water. Spritz around the places where evidence of mice is seen. Spray in rooms.

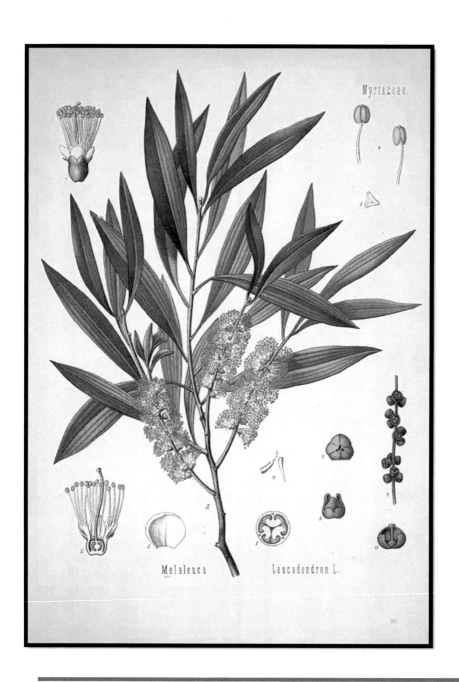

Myrtaceae.

Melaleuca   Leucadendron L.

(*Melaleuca alternifolia*)

Tea Tree essential oil is antiseptic. It is a strong antimicrobial that cleans up antibiotic resistant microbes from surfaces. It is also antifungal, antiviral, and anti-parasitic. Use it to treat insect bites, open wounds, and to repel biting insects.

It quickly penetrates tissue and can be applied on the skin to bring benefit to internal infections. Here at Joybilee Farm we treat milking does with hot, red lumps on their udders with tea tree oil in a salve. The tea tree penetrates the udder tissue and in most cases relieves the mastitis in a few days. It's one of the few things that can reach mastitis in the udder tissue.

TEA TREE

- Analgesic

- Antibacterial

- Antifungal

- Anti-inflammatory

- Anti-microbial

- Anti-parasitic

- Antiseptic

- Anti-viral

- Decongestant

- Deodorant

- Diaphoretic

- Expectorant

- Immune stimulant

- Insecticidal

- Vulnerary

Tea Tree adds a **middle note** to essential oil blends and perfumes.

USES OF TEA TREE ESSENTIAL OIL

TICK REPELLANT

Put 1 cup of rubbing alcohol, vodka, or cider vinegar and 1 tsp of tea tree essential oil in a spritz bottle. Shake well and spray the tops of your shoes, pant legs, and exposed skin. It will repel ticks and keep them from hanging on. We also use this to treat our llamas' legs, to keep the ticks from grabbing on as they graze in the long grass.

Warning: Don't use it on dogs, cats, or rabbits though. Pets will lick their legs and feet. They lack the liver enzymes to break down tea tree essential oil and it can cause toxicity and even death.

ITCH BE GONE

Use a cotton ball to apply to insect bites and stings to reduce inflammation, decrease itching, and prevent bacterial infection. Children and sensitive people should use 1 tsp. of carrier oil per drop of tea tree essential oil.

TICK REMOVAL

Apply 1 drop of tea tree essential oil on the backside of tick. It will kill the tick and make removal easier.

DISINFECTANT AND CLEANER

Add tea tree essential oil to your all-purpose cleaner and disinfectant to kill germs and make clean up easier.

GOO REMOVER

Use tea tree oil neat on chewing gum, sticky tree sap, or glue to remove the residue from hair, clothing, skin, or wood surfaces. It may remove the finish on some wood surfaces, so test in an inconspicuous area first.

WART REMOVER

Use 1 drop of tea tree essential oil on a wart on your hands or feet. Cover with a bandage and keep the area dry for at least 1 hour. Repeat twice a day until the wart falls off.

Tea Tree essential oil is a very effective antimicrobial to combat tooth abscesses and gum infections. While not a substitute for professional dental care, rubbing one drop of tea tree oil along the gum, and around the infected area, can buy you some time, when you are dealing with a painful abscess.

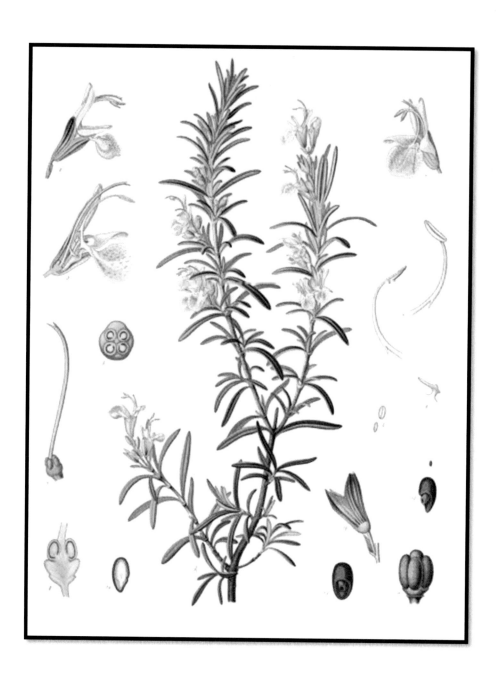

(Rosmarinus officinalis)

"Rosemary for remembrance." Rosemary is the herb for sharpened memory and for love. It is sharply balsamic and menthol in scent and provides a middle note to blends. It should be diluted with a carrier oil before use.

Rosemary is pain relieving, anti-arthritic, and anti-rheumatic. It is antispasmodic, antibacterial, antifungal, antioxidant, antiseptic, decongestant, and expectorant. It helps to break a fever. It helps normalize blood pressure. It is restorative, stimulant, and tonic. It supports the liver and aids digestion. It is astringent, tonifies tissue, and helps with painful menstrual periods. And it is considered an aphrodisiac.

Rosemary is a good essential oil to infuse in the room when you are creating, writing, or doing any activity that requires concentration. Do you have a late night study session, or a paper due in the morning? Infuse rosemary essential oil to help you remain alert and to aid in concentration and memory.

Rosemary is analgesic. Add it to a massage oil or arthritis salve to ease sore muscles or warm a sore back. It is also antifungal and antiseptic, making it idea to add with peppermint to a foot soak for achy feet.

- Analgesic

- Antibacterial

- Antifungal

- Antioxidant

- Anti-parasitic

- Anti-rheumatic

- Antiseptic

- Anti-spasmodic

- Aphrodisiac

- Astringent

- Carminative

- Cholagogue

- Cordial

- Decongestant

- Diaphoretic

- Digestive

- Diuretic

- Emmenagogue

- Expectorant

- Hepatic

- Hypertensive

- Nervine

- Restorative

- Rubefacient

- Stimulant

- Stomachic

- Sudorific

- Tonic

- Vulnerary

Rosemary is a **middle note** in blends.

USES FOR ROSEMARY ESSENTIAL OIL

PRE-EXERCISE MUSCLE WARM UP

1 tsp coconut oil plus 1 drop of rosemary essential oil, massage into your large muscles before exercise to stimulate circulation and increase warmth in order to reduce injuries.

STUDY AID

Diffuse 6 drops of rosemary essential oil in a room diffuser to increase alertness, and facilitate memory during study periods.

EASE MENSTRUAL PAIN

Massage 1 tsp of calendula infused oil and 1 drop of rosemary essential oil into your abdomen to relieve congestion and menstrual discomfort. Calendula infused oil stimulates lymph flow to ease the bloated feeling.

NO MORE DANDRUFF HAIR RINSE

Add 5 drops of rosemary essential oil to 1 cup of vinegar to rinse your hair after shampoo and conditioner. Rosemary will remove soap residue and leave your hair fresh and clean.

BACK PAIN

In 1 tbsp. of carrier oil add 10 drops of rosemary, 3 drops of peppermint, 5 drops of eucalyptus, and 5 drops of geranium essential oil. Massage into lower back to relieve discomfort and inflammation.

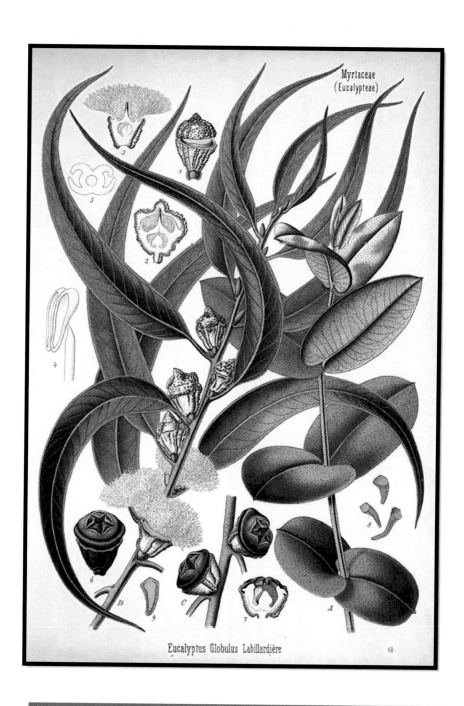

Eucalyptus Globulus Labillardière.

Myrtaceae
(Eucalypteae)

40

(*Eucalyptus sp.*)

Eucalyptus is a wakeup call. It is strongly menthol and is the scent most commonly associated with vapour rubs and cold remedies. It clears the sinuses and relieves chest and sinus congestion. It is a strong disinfectant and deodorizer and is a common ingredient in household cleaning products, laundry products, and cold remedies.

Eucalyptus is pain relieving, antibacterial, antifungal, anti-arthritic, and antiseptic. It relieves nerve pain, and is anti-spasmodic. It helps during colds and flu because it is anti-viral, and decongestant. It relieves a fever, and helps make a cough more productive. Eucalyptus blends well with peppermint and tea tree in blends formulated to relieve an unproductive cough and open the breathing. Eucalyptus is a good addition to muscle rubs, where pain relief and increased circulation is beneficial.

CAUTION:

There are several different essential oils labelled as Eucalyptus. All have strong decongestant and expectorant qualities. They vary in the percentage of ketones. Since ketones can be problematic for children under 10 and pregnant women, *Eucalyptus dives*, and *E. globulus* should not be used for children under 10 and pregnant women. *E. polybractea* is safe and is recommended for room diffusers, where pregnant women and young children are present. *Eucalyptus radiata* is safe for everyone. When purchasing your essential oils, the variety should be listed on the label to help you make an informed choice.

However, while noting this caution, understand that eucalyptus essential oil has been used for decades to ease cough and cold symptoms in all age groups. I have memories of my mother putting Vicks™ in the steam vaporizer in my bedroom in the 1960s. It was used to ease croup in young babies.

EUCALYPTUS

- Analgesic
- Antibacterial
- Antifungal
- Anti-inflammatory
- Anti-parasitic
- Anti-rheumatic
- Antiseptic
- Anti-spasmodic
- Anti-viral
- Decongestant
- Deodorant
- Depurative

- Diuretic

- Expectorant

- Febrifuge

- Insecticide

- Nervine

- Stimulant

- Vulnerary

Eucalyptus adds a **top note** to essential oil blends and perfumes.

USES FOR EUCALYPTUS ESSENTIAL OIL

EUCALYPTUS WOOL WASH

Add 20 drops of eucalyptus essential oil to the final rinse water when washing wool socks, sweaters, shawls, hats, or mittens. Eucalyptus repels wool moths and conditions wool.

EUCALYPTUS CHEST RUB

1 tbsp. cocoa butter
1 tbsp. sweet almond oil
6 drops of eucalyptus essential oil

Melt cocoa butter and sweet almond oil together over low heat. Blend well and allow the carrier oils to cool slightly. Add essential oils and stir well. Place in a well capped jar.

To use apply to the chest, the back, or the bottoms of the feet to relieve achy muscles, chest congestion, fever, and stuffy nose.

Use cautiously with children under 10, pregnant and nursing mothers. **See the caution above.**

REPEL FLEAS

Eucalyptus should not be sprayed directly on pets. However, a collar to which a few drops of eucalyptus essential oil has been applied, will repel fleas for several days. Reapply the eucalyptus essential oil to the collar, as necessary to maintain protection.

ROOM FRESHENER

Diffuse 4 drops eucalyptus essential oil in a room diffuser to cleanse the air, and combat viruses and microbes. It will make breathing easier and relieve the stuffy, clogged feeling in your sinuses and the scratchy feeling in your throat.

SHOWER PUCK FOR COLDS AND CONGESTION

Add 15 drops of eucalyptus, 1 tsp. of citric acid, and 1 tbsp. of baking soda to a bowl. Mix together and press into a silicone candy mold. Allow to harden overnight. Place on the floor of the shower stall during a hot shower. As the shower puck dissolves in the steam, eucalyptus will remove sluggishness from your brain, increase alertness, and loosen sinuses and chest congestion.

NOTES:

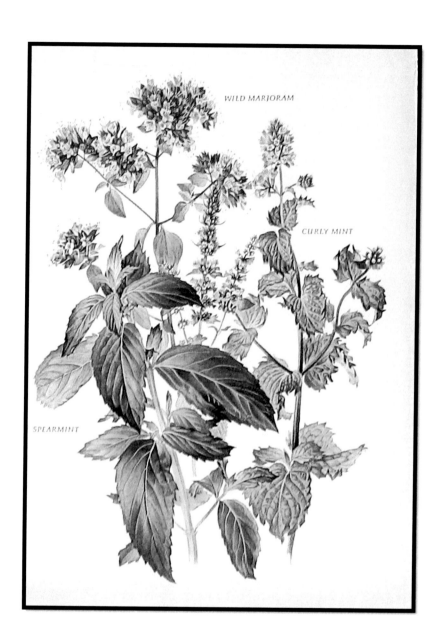

(*Origanum majorana*)

Sweet marjoram has a pleasant floral scent. It is anti-microbial, anti-viral, and anti-fungal like tea tree. Schnaublet notes in his book, *Advanced Aromatherapy*, that marjoram is noted for its healing virtue in whooping cough and acute bronchitis. It can be used interchangeably with tea tree oil, for those who dislike tea tree oil's strong scent. Use it in place of oregano oil with colds and bronchial congestion.

MARJORAM

- Analgesic

- Antioxidant

- Antiseptic

- Anti-spasmodic

- Anti-viral

- Carminative

- Cephalic

- Diaphoretic

- Digestive

- Diuretic

- Emmenagogue

- Expectorant

- Nervine

- Sedative

- Tonic

- Vasodilator

- Vulnerary

Marjoram is a **middle note** in essential oil blends and perfumes.

USES FOR MARJORAM ESSENTIAL OIL

USE INSTEAD OF LAVENDER

For those who are sensitive to lavender essential oil, marjoram is a good substitute.

RELAXING

Diffuse 4 drops of marjoram essential oil in a room diffuser to promote relaxation, and calm and relieve anxiety.

RELIEVE TENSION HEADACHE

Place ½ tsp of a carrier oil in your palm and add 2 drops of marjoram essential oil in your palm to make a 4% dilution. Rub your palms together to blend. Apply to your temples and the back of your neck to reduce tension and relieve a tension headache.

RELIEVE PMS SYMPTOMS

Place 1 drop of marjoram essential oil in a handkerchief and breathe deeply, inhaling the scent, when you feel hormonal stress and anxiety.

RELIEF OF BRONCHIAL SPASMS AND COUGHING

Place 1 tbsp. of sweet almond oil or coconut oil in an amber glass bottle. Add 3 drops of marjoram essential oil. Shake to mix well. Take 1 drop of this mixture under your tongue and allow it to absorb in your mouth, to relieve sore throat, bronchial spasm, and unproductive coughing.

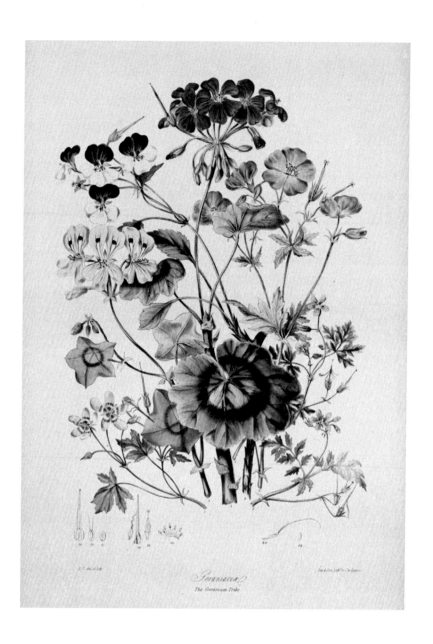

Geraniaceæ
The Geranium Tribe.

(*Pelargonium odorantissimum*)

Geranium smells differently to different people. It also reacts differently to different people. It is calming to some, stimulating to others, and to some antiseptic smelling. It is anti-fungal without upsetting the microbial balance or harming good bacteria. It is hormone balancing. For those who dislike the scent of lavender essential oil, geranium can be used interchangeably.

Apply 1 drop of geranium essential oil with 1 tsp. of carrier oil to make a 1% dilution and massage it over the abdomen during menses to relieve menstrual cramps and discomfort.

Geranium is a good oil to diffuse in a room if you expect to have a conflict. It is balancing and grounding. Geranium oil calms without being overwhelming. It is especially valuable for skin care. Rose geranium oil is also insect repellent. When used in a blend, you don't need very much geranium oil. Use it sparingly.

GERANIUM

- Analgesic

- Antibacterial

- Anti-depressant,

- Anti-diabetic

- Anti-inflammatory

- Anti-parasitic
- Antiseptic
- Astringent
- Cicatrisant
- Deodorant
- Diuretic
- Emmenagogue
- Hepatic
- Hormone modulator
- Insecticide
- Regenerative
- Rubefacient
- Sedative
- Styptic
- Tonic
- Vasoconstrictor

Geranium essential oil brings a **middle note** to essential oil blends and perfumes.

USES FOR GERANIUM ESSENTIAL OIL

INSECT REPELLANT

Geranium essential oil repels mosquitoes and biting insects. Use 3 drops in 1 tbsp. of carrier oil and apply to face and exposed skin. It has a strong rose scent.

FACEMASK

Use 1 tsp. of French green clay and make a paste with 1 tbsp. of water. Add 2 drops of geranium essential oil. Stir well. Apply to face, avoiding eyes, nostrils, and mouth. Allow to dry and rinse off. This stimulates circulation while it exfoliates and tightens up loose skin.

AFTER SHAVE

Blend together 1 cup of witch hazel, 3 drops of geranium essential oil, and 1 tsp of jojoba oil in a glass bottle. Shake well to blend. Splash on as an after shave to reduce redness, and stop bleeding. Pat dry. Follow with moisturizer.

TO TREAT BLEEDING AND WOUNDS

Add a drop of geranium essential oil to a splash of colloidal silver on a bandaid. The geranium oil is astringent and styptic and will help the blood vessels to tighten and the bleeding to stop. It is also antimicrobial and with the colloidal silver will prevent infection.

HOMEMADE ROSE GERANIUM DEODORANT

10 drops of rose geranium essential oil, 3 tbsp. coconut oil, 2 tbsp. cocoa butter, 2 tbsp. baking soda, 1 tbsp. tapioca starch. Melt the coconut oil and the cocoa butter together over low heat. Stir in baking soda and starch. Cool until blood warm. Stir in essential oil. Press into roll-up deodorant container or store in a small glass jar. Use as you would any deodorant.

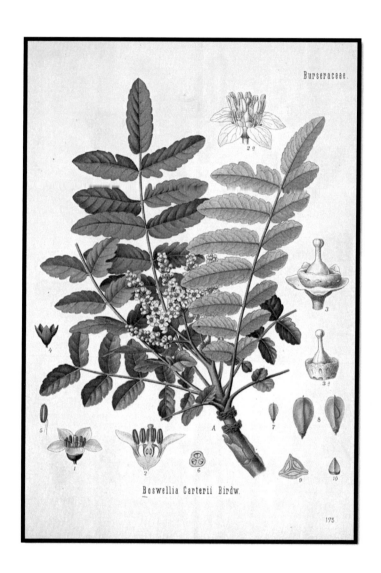

Burseraceae.

Boswellia Carterii Birdw.

175

(*Boswellia carteri*)

Frankincense is precious oil made from the resin of a Middle Eastern tree. It is a potent immune strengthener. Scientific studies are showing promise as a treatment for ovarian cancer. It is a mood elevator.

FRANKINCENSE

- Analgesic
- Antifungal
- Anti-inflammatory
- Anti-microbial
- Antioxidant
- Antiseptic
- Astringent
- Carminative
- Digestive
- Diuretic
- Expectorant
- Sedative
- Tonic

- Vulnerary

Frankincense brings a **bass note** to essential oil blends and perfumes.

USES FOR FRANKINCENSE ESSENTIAL OIL

ANTI-AGING SERUM

Mix 1 tbsp. rosehip oil, 1 tbsp. argon oil, 2 drops of frankincense essential oil, 1 drop of myrrh essential oil, 1/8th tsp. vitamin E. Mix this together in a 30 ml amber or cobalt glass bottle with a dropper lid. To use place a few drops on your finger and massage gently over face, paying close attention to the delicate skin around your eyes and mouth. Applying it here is where it will do you the most good. This is rich in antioxidants and removes the appearance of fine lines, making your skin more supple and elastic, while it moisturizes.

FACIAL STEAM

Add 2 to 4 drops of frankincense essential oil to a bowl of steaming water (not too hot. Don't get burnt). Place a towel over your head and breathe deeply of the steam and allow it to open your pores. Breathe deeply for 15 minutes. Close your pores with a splash of cold water and finish your facial with a splash of rose hydrosol.

OWIE SPRAY

½ cup witch hazel, 5 drops of frankincense essential oil, 5 drops of lavender essential oil, and 5 drops of myrrh essential oil. Place all the ingredients in an amber glass bottle with a spray mister top. To use this antibacterial, soothing spray, spritz on the wound to clean and disinfect. Allow to dry naturally. Cover wound with a bandage to keep clean.

MENSTRUAL PAIN

Massage 1 tsp. of jojoba oil and 3 drops of frankincense essential oil into the abdomen during menses to relieve pain and congestion.

CALMING AND CENTERING

Place 4 drops of frankincense essential oil in a room diffuser to bring calm and focus to your mood.

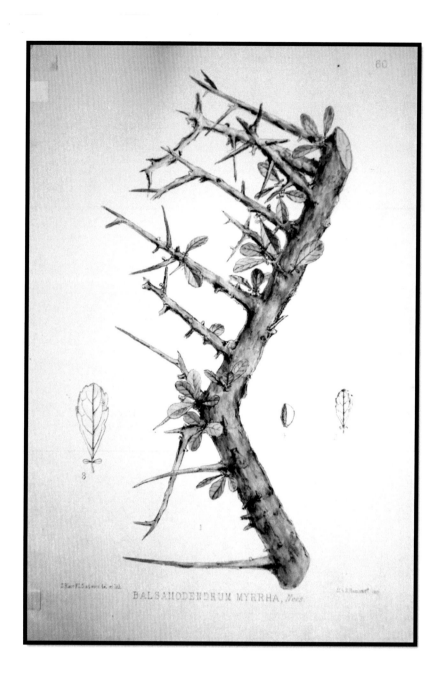

BALSAMODENDRUM MYRRHA, *Nees*

(*Commiphora molmol*)

Myrrh is another resinous precious oil. It is antiseptic, anti-viral, and anti-inflammatory. It is often used in dental care and skin care. While it is an expensive essential oil a very little goes a long way. It is a fixative for other scents and is a base note. When used in a blend, myrrh will linger.

The essential oil is thick and may clog the dropper on your essential oil bottle. Don't buy it in large quantities, as it has a propensity to dry in the bottle if it is stored a long time.

MYRRH

- Anti-catarrhal

- Antifungal

- Anti-inflammatory

- Anti-microbial

- Antiseptic

- Anti-spasmodic

- Antiviral

- Astringent

- Carminative

- Cicatrisant

- Emmenagogue

- Expectorant

- Fungicidal

- Sedative

- Stomachic

- Tonic

- Uterine Tonic

- Vulnerary

Myrrh offers a **base note** in essential oil blends and perfumes. It is also a fixative for other more volatile oils like citrus, making them last a little longer in the blend.

USES FOR MYRRH ESSENTIAL OIL

ANTISEPTIC MOUTHWASH AND GARGLE

1 cup of warm water, ¼ tsp. Himalayan salt, and 2 drops of myrrh essential oil. Mix together and use as a daily gargle and mouthwash. It will cleanse and heal gum pain, and remove bacteria that causes dental disease, while it tightens tissue and eases pain.

SWEET ORANGE AND MYRRH PERFUME BLEND

Myrrh is a fixative for perfume blends strengthening the longevity of the top note. Perfume blends that contain citrus oils are especially helped when myrrh is added in the blend. Create a solid perfume by blending together 1 tbsp. jojoba oil, 1 tsp. sweet almond oil, 2 tsp. cocoa butter. Heat together in a double boiler until cocoa butter is melted and all the oils are blended together. Stir in ½ tsp. sweet orange essential oil, ¼ tsp. myrrh essential oil, ¼ tsp. frankincense essential oil. Pour into 1 ounce tin. Label. Use it as you would any perfume.

FRENCH GREEN CLAY MASK

In a small dish mix 1 tbsp. rose hydrosol, 2 tsp. French green clay, 4 drops of myrrh essential oil, and 2 drops of rosemary essential oil. Mix the clay into the hydrosol, but only use as much of the clay as you need to get the consistency of vanilla pudding. If it's too thick, add a little water, ½ tsp at a time until it's the right consistency. Add the essential oils. Mix well.

To apply pull your hair back. Apply to your face, but avoid eyes and mucus membranes. Allow to dry about 20 minutes. Wash off with tepid water. Pat dry. Apply moisturizer such as the **anti-aging serum** recipe (p. 75).

Clay is toning and astringent. It will increase circulation and tighten pores, while it exfoliates. Your face will be red when you are done. Don't use this mask right before a date or important occasion. It takes about 4 to 6 hours before the circulation in your face returns to normal and you lose that red-heat in your cheeks. The best time to apply it is the day before a special occasion when you need to look your best.

ANTI-INFLAMMATORY MASSAGE OIL

Mix together in a small jar, 1 tbsp. sweet almond oil and 3 drops of myrrh essential oil. Massage as usual.

OIL PULLING TABS FOR DENTAL HYGIENE

¼ c. coconut oil, 10 drops of myrrh essential oil. Soften coconut oil. Stir in myrrh essential oil and blend well. Line a baking sheet with parchment paper. Drop by 1 tsp. onto baking sheet. Place in freezer until solid. Package this in a glass jar. Keep refrigerated. Use one for oil pulling each morning to improve oral health. (Yield: 12 tabs)

Now that you have met some essential oils, it's time to get to know them better. The following recipes use these top 10 beginner essential oils in easy recipes to allow you to quickly gain experience using them. Get to know their scents, their actions and most of all the way they make you feel.

Do they relax you or energize you? Do they relieve pain or stimulate? Are they toning and astringent or do they loosen and calm? Not everyone reacts to each essential oil in the same way. Your constitution is different than mine.

Keep notes about your personal experiences. This will help to guide you in your choices of essential oils and allow you to tweak each recipe to make it the very best it can be for you and your family. There are extra pages at the end of each section for you to record your own experiences, as well as a place to add your own personal recipes.

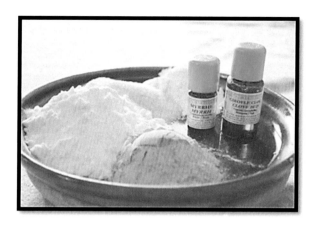

REMINERALIZING TOOTH POWDER

This tooth powder is the culmination of 20 years of experimenting with non-commercial toothpaste alternatives. It remineralizes, reduces bacteria, and strengthens and tonifies gums and soft tissue in the mouth, reducing pain and inflammation. While not a substitute for seeing your dental professional, it is a home remedy that is within reach of everyone.

INGREDIENTS:
3 tbsp. calcium carbonate
2 tbsp. bentonite clay
1/2 cup baking soda
1/4 cup Himalayan salt, whirled in your spice grinder until a fine powder
1 tsp. peppermint eo
10 drops myrrh eo,
10 drops tea tree eo

This tooth powder has no fillers. Every part is essential. Initially buying the ingredients may seem expensive, but it will give you many months of dental hygiene for your efforts.

Use glass, or wood to mix this tooth powder. Bentonite is reactive to metal. Mix calcium, clay, baking soda, and Himalayan salt in a glass bowl. Blend it thoroughly. Add peppermint eo, myrrh eo, and clove eo and mix well. Divide between two 4 oz. glass jars. Cap tightly.

To use: Moisten toothbrush with water and dip into the powder. Brush as you would brush with toothpaste. Spit out the mixture when you are done brushing your teeth. Do not swallow. Rinse with warm water.

PEPPERMINT FOOT BUTTER

Refreshing, antibacterial, and analgesic, peppermint foot butter helps soothe rough, cracked winter feet. This takes advantage of the antimicrobial actions of peppermint and rosemary, and the cooling sensation of peppermint to invigorate your tired feet.

INGREDIENTS:
4 oz. cocoa butter
½ c. organic coconut oil
8 drops of peppermint essential oil
4 drops of rosemary essential oil

METHOD:

In a saucepan, melt cocoa butter and coconut oil together until just melted. Allow to cool slightly. Add essential oils. Stir well. Pour into 2 4oz. glass jars. Seal. Allow to harden.

Use this after a bath or shower, where the oil will lock the moisture into your feet.

ORANGE LIP BALM

With the bright, cheering scent and sweet taste of orange and the skin rejuvenating actions of calendula infused oil, this lip balm will refresh as well as moisturize. Stop buying petroleum based lip balms and use this natural, healthy alternative that you can make yourself.

INGREDIENTS:
1 tsp. beeswax
1 tbsp. coconut oil
1 tbsp. calendula infuse olive oil
1/8th tsp. vitamin E oil
8 drops orange EO
2 lip balm tubes

METHOD:

Melt beeswax, coconut oil, and calendula infused olive oil together. Stir in vitamin E oil as a preservative. Allow to cool slightly. Add 8 drops of orange essential oil. Pour into 2 balm tubes.

PEPPERMINT PATTY LIP BALM

Another great tasting, refreshing lip balm to lock in moisture and keep your lips from chapping in the wind and sun.

INGREDIENTS:
1 tbsp. organic cocoa butter
1 tbsp. coconut oil
1 tsp. calendula infuse olive oil
1/8th tsp. vitamin E oil
8 drops peppermint EO
2 lip balm tubes

METHOD:

Melt cocoa butter, coconut oil, and calendula infused olive oil together. Stir in vitamin E oil as a preservative. Allow to cool slightly. Add 8 drops of peppermint essential oil. Pour into 2 balm tubes.

DIY LAVENDER BODY SCRUB

Exfoliating, relaxing, and moisturizing, while it stimulates lymph drainage and increases circulation. Try this quick to make salt scrub that uses lavender and rosemary essential oils to relax and soothe.

INGREDIENTS:
1 cup Dead Sea salts
1 cup organic extra-virgin coconut oil
15 drops of lavender essential oil
5 drops of rosemary essential oil

METHOD:

Mix all ingredients in a wide mouth pint jar. Stir well.

CUTICLE SUGAR SCRUB

Moisturizing, exfoliating, and extra rich for dry, damaged skin and brittle nails. Argon oil and pomegranate oil are excellent moisturizers for aging skin, rich in antioxidants. Myrrh and frankincense essential oils are good for the skin and the nails, with long lasting antimicrobial and antifungal actions. Use this after a bath, and before you go to bed to strengthen nails and soften cuticles.

INGREDIENTS:

½ cup of organic sugar
1 tbsp. argon oil
1 tbsp. pomegranate oil
¼ cup of extra-virgin coconut oil
5 drops of myrrh essential oil
5 drops of frankincense essential oil
10 drops of orange essential oil

METHOD:

Mix sugar and oils together. Add the essential oils and mix well. Put in a 4 oz. wide mouth jar with a tight fitting lid. Use to scrub hands, and especially cuticles to exfoliate, soften, and moisturize. Rinse hands with warm water and pat dry. Apply nail polish as usual.

RELAXING BATH SALTS

Dead Sea salts are rich in magnesium and trace minerals that are easily absorbed through the skin. Lavender essential oil is relaxing and uplifting, while geranium essential oil helps to balance hormones, relieving pelvic congestion, and calming mood swings and anxiety.

INGREDIENTS:

1 cup baking soda
1 cup Dead Sea salt
1 tbsp. coconut oil
7 drops lavender
5 drops geranium

METHOD:

Stir together the essential oils and coconut oil. When it is thoroughly combined, stir in the salts. Store in a tightly sealed jar. To use add ½ to 1 cup of bath salts to a tub of hot water. Soak for a minimum of 20 minutes to maximize the relaxing and detoxifying effects.

DEAD SEA MUD MASK

The minerals in the Dead Sea have been used for millennium to bring health and beauty to royalty. Cleopatra had a health spa at the Dead Sea and used its mud and salt to enhance her feminine beauty. Today tourists to Israel cover their bodies in the mud to get the analgesic, relaxing, and tonic results that the Dead Sea is famous for. You can get Dead Sea mud online from several sources for this easy mud mask. See **my sources** *at the end of the book. Don't just use it on your face, make a big batch and plaster it on wherever you need a bit of extra minerals, detoxification, and pain relief.*

INGREDIENTS:
1 ½ tsp. Dead Sea mud
1 tbsp. water
1 tsp. bentonite clay
5 drops myrrh essential oil
2 drops of rosemary essential oil
2 drops of lavender essential oil

METHOD:

Mix Dead Sea mud and clay until thoroughly blended. Add essential oils for their purifying, balancing, and antimicrobial actions. Use within 5 days of blending.

TO APPLY THE FACIAL MASK:

Pull back your hair. Ring out a face cloth in hot water and place on your face to open your pores. Hold for a few seconds. Remove wash cloth and while face is still damp apply the mask, avoiding the eye area. Apply using your fingers in a circular motion. Apply as thickly as you like, being sure that you've covered your face. **Avoid the delicate skin around your eyes**.

Now go read a book, weed the garden, or make a cup of tea. Allow the mask to dry completely. About 20 to 30 minutes should do, depending on how warm and dry your home is.

You'll use about 1/2 tsp. of this mask. Place a lid on the jar and keep the mask in the fridge. It should keep for up to two weeks in the fridge. You can use this mask once or twice a week. More often if you have a break out of acne. It increases circulation and detoxifies.

RINSE OFF THE MASK:

To rinse off the mask, use a face cloth dipped in warm water. Get every last bit of the mask off. And then rinse your face with warm water. Pat your face dry. Your skin should feel tighter and smoother. It may feel hot for a few hours. Don't be concerned. This is a normal response to a face mask. It increases circulation and helps to remove impurities from the skin. After a few hours your skin will return to normal.

Apply **anti-aging serum** (p. 75) to your whole face to complete the facial pampering. Your skin will drink it in.

DEAD SEA MUD AND SILK FACIAL MASK

Silk protein lightens the heaviness of the Dead Sea mud in this facial mask. Silk also attracts moisture to your skin, leaving your skin smooth and supple, while it tightens your pores, exfoliates, and nourishes.

INGREDIENTS:
1½ tsp Dead Sea mud
1 tbsp. water
¼ tsp silk protein powder
1 tbsp. French green clay (or other natural clay)
5 drops myrrh essential oil
1 drop rose geranium essential oil
3 drops frankincense essential oil

METHOD:

Place the Dead Sea mud and water together in a small jar and mix together to dilute the mud. Stir in the silk protein, and then stir in the French green clay, a little bit at a time. Stir well till the mask is smooth and creamy. Add the myrrh, rose geranium, and frankincense essential oils and stir to combine. It should be the consistency of vanilla pudding. To thin it a bit add more water, a ¼ tsp. at a time, until the mask is the right consistency to apply.

TO APPLY THE FACIAL MASK:

Pull back your hair. Ring out a face cloth in hot water and place on your face to open your pores. Hold for a few seconds. Remove wash cloth and while face is still damp apply the mask, avoiding the eye area. Apply using your fingers in a circular motion. Apply as thickly as you like, being sure that you've covered your face. Avoid the delicate skin around your eyes.

Now go read a book, weed the garden, or make a cup of tea. Allow the mask to dry completely. About 20 to 30 minutes should do, depending on how warm and dry your home is.

You'll use about 1/2 tsp. of this mask. Place a lid on the jar and keep the mask in the fridge. It should keep for up to two weeks in the fridge. You can use this mask once or twice a week. More often if you have a break out.

RINSE OFF THE MASK

To rinse off the mask, use a face cloth dipped in warm water. Get every last bit of the mask off. And then rinse your face with warm water. Pat your face dry. Your skin should feel tighter and smoother.

Apply **anti-aging serum** (p. 75) to your whole face to complete the facial pampering. Your skin will drink it in.

MOISTURIZING SHAVING SOAP

This shaving soap is antimicrobial, rejuvenating the skin, and boosting the immune system while it moisturizes and provides a barrier between tender skin and the sharp blade.

INGREDIENTS:
1/4 cup coconut oil
1/4 cup soap, grated
2 tbsp. cocoa butter
2 tsp. baking soda
4 drops tea tree essential oil
4 drops of myrrh essential oil
4 drops of frankincense essential oil

METHOD:

Melt soap, cocoa butter, and coconut oil together so that they blend well. Add baking soda and whip with a hand blender until well blended. As it's mixing drop in essential oils and continue mixing until light and frothy. Spoon this into a 500 ml, wide mouth jar. Cap tightly.

Use with a shaving brush or rub a small amount between your hand to foam and apply to area prior to shaving. Use your razor as usual.

This section includes essential oil recipes for your first aid kit, to help you deal with minor cuts, abrasions, and other minor complaints. For serious illness, shortness of breath, chest pain, difficulty breathing, a high fever, or neck pain accompanied by fever, always consult with your personal medical practitioner.

BOOBOO OINTMENT

Calming, cooling, and antimicrobial, this ointment helps when kisses just aren't enough.

INGREDIENTS:
5 tbsp. bees' wax
2 tbsp. coconut oil
1/2 cup of infused calendula oil
6 drops of lavender essential oil
4 drops of peppermint essential oil
4 drops of tea tree essential oil

METHOD:

Melt beeswax and coconut oil together. Warm calendula infused oil and mix with beeswax mixture. Allow mixture to cool slightly. Add essential oils. Mix well.

Store in a 4 oz. glass jar with a tight lid.

To use on bruises, bumps, or scraps, wash wound and apply salve. Ointment is disinfectant and cooling.

CHEST RUB REMEDY

Better than the OTC chest rub that is made with petroleum, use **Eucalyptus radiata** *if you are making this for a child under 10 years of age. See the notes on* **Eucalyptus sp.**

INGREDIENTS:

2 tbsp. melted beeswax
6 tbsp. of coconut oil
10 drops of eucalyptus essential oil
3 drops of peppermint essential oil
5 drops of rosemary essential oil

METHOD:

Melt beeswax and coconut oil together. Allow to cool slightly. Add essential oils. Store in 4 oz. jar with tight lid. Rub on back and chest to loosen breathing and unclog sinuses. Cooling and analgesic on sore muscles, too.

NASAL INHALER FOR CHEST AND NASAL CONGESTION

You can make this antimicrobial salt inhaler to carry in your purse. Use an inhaler tube but remove the bleached cotton wick and replace with salt and essential oils.

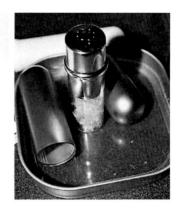

INGREDIENTS:

1/4 c. Dead Sea salt
5 drops eucalyptus essential oil
5 drops of peppermint essential oil
5 drops of rosemary essential oil

METHOD:

Mix salt and essential oils. Place ½ tsp into the well of a nasal inhaler. Cap. To use place the inhaler on nostril and breathe deeply. Hold your breath. Exhale. Repeat on the other side.

This mixture can also be used in a foot bath or a steam inhalation.

STEAM INHALATION

Use the above recipe

METHOD:

Place 2 tbsp. of the salt mixture into a bowl of very hot water – not so hot that it will burn you, though.

Place face over the steam and inhale. For deeper penetration, place head over bowl and under a towel. Breathe for 5 minutes. The salt is antiseptic and the essential oils will clear the sinus cavities.

FOOT BATH FOR RELIEF OF COLDS AND FLU SYMPTOMS

Use the above recipe

METHOD:

Place ¼ cup into a foot bath with hot water. Stir to dissolve. Soak feet in the foot bath for at least 20 minutes. Dry well and keep your feet warm to encourage circulation.

DIY DECONGESTANT INHALER 2

You'll be amazed at how quickly your sinuses and your thinking clear when you use this sinus decongestant. I keep one in my purse for those times when I feel groggy and tight in the middle of the day, and I have a long drive ahead of me.

INGREDIENTS:

½ cup of Dead Sea salt
5 ml eucalyptus
5 ml lavender essential oil
3 ml tea tree essential oil
20 drops rosemary essential oil
10 drops marjoram essential oil

DIRECTIONS:

Mix essential oils and Dead Sea salt thoroughly in a bowl. Place ½ tsp of the mixture into glass chamber of inhaler or into the plastic chamber of a disposable inhaler. Jiggle the salt gently and add more salt until no more salt can be added. Place the plug firmly into the bottom of the plastic inhaler to hold salt in place or place cap on the glass inhaler and insert the glass chamber into the protective steel base. Cap both inhalers tightly and label the plastic inhaler "for sinus congestion".

CALMING ROLL ON FOR KIDS

This is the magic tube. When the kids are sweaty, cranky, or excited roll this on the bottoms of their feet or on the inside of their elbows and watch the stress melt away.

INGREDIENTS:

1 tbsp. sweet almond oil
10 drops of sweet orange essential oil
10 drops of lavender essential oil
5 drops of marjoram essential oil
15 ml Amber roll-on bottle

METHOD:

Mix all ingredients in an amber bottle with a roll-on applicator. To use, apply to the bottoms of the feet.

IMMUNE BOOSTING TRAVEL INHALER

This will keep your nasal passages clean during long flights where the cabin air is recirculated, while it clears that queasy feeling from motion sickness.

INGREDIENTS:

1 Tbsp. Dead Sea salts
3 drops of myrrh essential oil
3 drops of frankincense essential oil
5 drops of lavender essential oil

3 drops of tea tree essential oil
3 drops of peppermint essential oil

Mix essential oils with salts. Place 1 tsp. into a glass inhaler tube. Pack in your carry-on luggage to sniff during long flights. It will keep your nose clear of bacteria and viruses. Helps with queasiness, too.

BUG REPELLENT FOR CHILDREN

Keep mosquitoes and biting flies away with this spray on bug spray. If using this with very young children infuse eucalyptus leaves and peppermint leaves with the witch hazel before making up the recipe. If you are using it for adults, you can substitute 10 drops each of peppermint and eucalyptus essential oils for the leaves, instead of infusing them in the witch hazel.

INGREDIENTS:
1 cup of witch hazel
¼ cup of peppermint leaves
¼ cup of eucalyptus leaves
5 drops of lavender essential oil
3 drops of geranium essential oil
3 drops of lemon essential oil

METHOD:

Infuse witch hazel with peppermint and eucalyptus leaves for 1 month, on a sunny window. Strain the witch hazel and discard the spent plant material. Add the essential oils to the witch hazel infusion and place in a spritz bottle. Spray skin and clothes, but avoid eyes. Re-spray as often as necessary to repel biting insects.

BUG BITE ROLL ON:

Those itchy bites make for crabby kids. Use this antimicrobial, anti-itch roll on to remove the sting, the swelling, and the itching.

INGREDIENTS.
2 Tbsp. sweet almond oil
12 drops of lavender essential oil
5 drops of tea tree essential oil
5 drops of myrrh essential oil

METHOD:

Place in 50 ml amber bottle with roller ball cap. To use roll onto bug bite as often as needed to remove itch and soothe. Giving each child their own roll on gives them some control over the relief.

COUGH AND COLD DETOX BATH

Lavender essential oil, eucalyptus, and sweet orange essential oil combine to open sinuses, sooth achy muscles, and boost the immune system to help you feel better fast.

INGREDIENTS:
3 cups Epsom salts

1 cup of baking soda
3 tbsp. coconut oil
12 drops of lavender essential oil
8 drops Eucalyptus essential oil
4 drops sweet orange essential oil

METHOD:

Combine the essential oils with the coconut oil and stir well to combine. Make sure that the essential oils are evenly dispersed throughout. Combine the oils with the salts and continue to stir until no lumps remain. Store this in an airtight container.

The coconut oil can make the bath tub slippery, so be extra cautious when getting in and out of the tub, when using this detox bath mixture.

TO USE:

For teens & adults: 1/2 cup of salts in a bath filled with warm water.

For children aged 7-12: 1/4 cup in a bath filled with warm water.

For children aged 2-6: 1-2 T into a bath with warm water.

Soak for 10-15 minutes or until clear breathing has been achieved.

COOLING LAVENDER SUNBURN BURN SPRAY

A cooling spray for when it hurts too much to touch. Just a spritz will bring cooling relief and start the herbal rejuvenation. Both lavender and aloe vera are traditionally used for minor burns. The tannins in green tea are cooling, astringent, and pain relieving.

INGREDIENTS:

1 cup of strong green tea, cooled
¼ c. aloe vera gel
12 drops of lavender essential oil

METHOD:

Put the green tea and aloe in a bottle and shake well to completely mix. Add the lavender essential oil. Shake before using. Spritz on sunburned skin or on minor burns to cool. Use immediately to quench the fire of a burn. For extra cooling, keep this in the fridge or an ice chest and spritz on as often as needed.

Don't use on a major burn – instead get immediate medical help.

Apply your new knowledge and experience with essential oils and replace those toxic commercial cleaners with a healthy natural product. You'll reduce your packaging waste and create an oasis in your home with these easy to make recipes.

TOILET BOWL CLEANER

This is one of the toughest places in the house to keep clean, especially if you live in an area with hard water. This nontoxic mixture sanitizes while it loosens tough mineral deposits. Get the citric acid where you buy canning supplies or spices.

INGREDIENTS:
¼ c. citric acid
¼ c. baking soda
15 drops of orange or lemon essential oil

METHOD:

Mix orange oil and citric acid together. Drop into toilet. Allow to sit for 15 minutes. Add baking soda. Wait for the fizzing to cease. Scrub with a toilet brush and flush.

BASIN, TUB, AND TILE CLEANER

Toss the foaming cleaner. It isn't foam that cleans the grout and the soap scum. This easy to use natural cleaner deodorizes, removes soap scum, and has a mild abrasive action to get deep into the corners where bacteria hide. *It's antimicrobial and will leave behind the fresh scent of lemon-tea tree essential oil.*

INGREDIENTS:

1 cup of baking soda
¼ cup of bentonite clay
½ cup of grated soap (leftover soap works well for this)
15 drops of tea tree essential oil
5 drops of lemon essential oil

METHOD.

Add all the ingredients to a food processor and process until the soap is broken up and the mixture looks like fine powder. Put it in a jar with a shaker top. Use in the place of powdered cleaners to clean sinks, tubs, and bathroom fixtures. It has a bit of gritty cleaning power, disinfects, and whitens.

SHOWER CLEANER

Put in a spray bottle. Use once a day to clean the shower and keep it fresh smelling. A little daily exercise saves a lot of time each week.

INGREDIENTS:

1 cup vinegar
1/4 cup vodka
1/2 cup water
20 drops lemon oil
10 drops eucalyptus oil

METHOD:

Place all ingredients in a spray bottle and shake well. Store the bottle in the shower and spray the entire shower daily after each use. A little clean up every day saves time.

WINDOW AND MIRROR CLEANER

Easy to make and no need to polish to remove streaks. If you want it to look like the commercial product add a drop or two of blue liquid food colouring.

INGREDIENTS:
1 cup of vinegar
¼ cup of vodka
2 cups of water
10 drops of lemon oil

METHOD:

Mix all ingredients in a spray bottle. Shake well. Use to clean windows and mirrors.

DIY DUSTER POLISH

Like the lemon duster polish with the TV commercial, but this one is nontoxic and won't stress your lungs when you use it.

INGREDIENTS:
⅓ cup water

1 tablespoon liquid castile soap
20 drops sweet orange essential oil
10 drops eucalyptus essential oil
10 drops lemon essential oil
4 oz. spray bottle with fine mister

METHOD:

Mix all ingredients into an amber glass bottle with a fine spray mister. Cap and shake well.

To use: Spray dust cloth and wipe to dust furniture. For best results use an old wool sock in need of darning. Wool is naturally electrostatic and will attract dust particles to itself without the need of scrubbing.

WOOD POLISH FOR WOODEN CUTTING BOARDS

Keep your wooden spoons, kraut pounders, spurtles, and cutting boards conditioned and clean with this easy to make, food safe, wood polish. It cleans and protects.

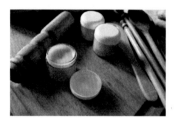

INGREDIENTS:

2 tbsp. beeswax
4 tbsp. walnut oil
1 tbsp. coconut oil
20 drops of sweet orange oil

METHOD:

Melt beeswax in a tin can. When its fully melted warm up walnut oil and coconut oil and mix together with melted bees wax. When fully blended, allow it to cool slightly. Add sweet orange oil. Put in 3 2oz. Glass jars and cap tightly.

To use wipe the polish generously on clean wooden cutting boards, wooden spoons, wooden kraut pounders and other wooden utensils. Allow the polish to permeate the wood for 30 minutes. Wipe off the excess polish with a dry cloth. Buff to clean and shine.

LEMON ALL-PURPOSE ANTI-MICROBIAL CLEANER

This all-purpose cleaner will leave your home with a lemon-fresh scent, while it cleans and sanitizes.

INGREDIENTS:
1 ½ cup of white vinegar
¼ cup of vodka
1 tsp. liquid castile soap
1 tsp. lemon essential oil
¼ tsp. tea tree essential oil
¼ tsp. eucalyptus essential oil

METHOD:

Put all the ingredients in a 500 ml spray bottle. Label. Shake well before using. Use as you would any disinfectant spray cleaner.

ANTIBACTERIAL WIPES

Use these instead of the commercial wipes to clean hands, cart handles, and door knobs, when you are out and about. Don't bring the germs home.

INGREDIENTS:
1/4 cup of vinegar or vodka
1 tsp. tea tree essential oil
1 tsp. lavender essential oil
1 tsp. eucalyptus essential oil
1/2 tsp. lemon essential oil
1/2 tsp. rosemary essential oil
A roll of paper towels

METHOD:

Take the paper towels and cut each paper towel in quarters, separating the towels on the perforation. Take the towels and roll each one up in a single roll, being sure that the new towel is added under the flap of the one that went before it. In this way, as you remove a towel from the roll, another towel will come up to take its place, like the way a tissue box works.

Keep cutting paper towels into quarters and rolling them in this way, until your roll of paper towels fits snugly into your jar.

In a separate cup measure the vinegar (or vodka), and the essential oils. Drizzle the vinegar mixture over the top of the paper towels inside the jar. Put on the lid and shake the jar. Allow to sit undisturbed for at least 15 minutes. The dry paper towels will wick-up the excess moisture. You can leave any extra liquid in the jar or pour it off when all the paper towels are uniformly damp.

To use, remove the outermost paper towel from the bundle in the jar. This will bring the next wipe to the top of the jar for the next person to use. Keep the jar capped tightly when not in use.

I keep a jar of antibacterial wipes in the Herbal First Aid Kit, and a jar in each vehicle. It's come in handy several times, especially in winter when there are so many colds and flu going around.

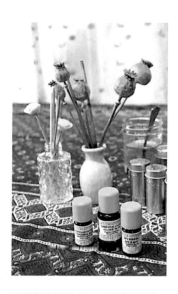

HOLIDAY DIFFUSER BLEND

That sweet Christmas fragrance can warm your home with this diffuser blend that reminds you of oranges, and incense. As a bonus, these essential oils will keep the air clean and remove bacteria and viruses, too.

INGREDIENTS:

½ cup carrier oil, sweet almond oil, olive oil,

¼ tsp. vitamin e oil

½ tsp. frankincense essential oil

½ tsp. myrrh essential oil

½ tsp. sweet orange essential oil

½ tsp. marjoram essential oil

METHOD:

Prepare bamboo skewers, reeds, or natural diffuser stems by cutting to 6 inch length with sharp scissors or pruning shears. Clean off any debris. If you want to buy reed diffuser sticks rather than gather them from the wild, you can get them at Amazon or a Mountain Rose Herbs. See **sources**.

In a 1 cup mason jar mix carrier oil, of your choice, with the essential oils. The carrier oil should have a neutral smell and remain stable at room temperature, such as sweet almond oil or grapeseed oil. This combination of essential oils gives a complex fragrance that lingers.

- Analgesic – relieves pain

- Antibacterial – inhibits the growth and replication of bacteria

- Anti-catarrhal – dries mucus and aids in removing it from the body

- Anti-depressant – elevates mood

- Anti-diabetic – aids in stabilizing blood sugar

- Anti-emetic – reduces the incidence and severity of nausea and vomiting

- Antifungal – inhibits the growth and replication of fungi

- Anti-inflammatory – soothes inflammation and directly reduces the inflammatory response in tissue

- Anti-microbial – inhibits the growth and replication of microbes

- Anti-neuralgic – relieves or reduces nerve pain

- Antioxidant – prevents free radical stressor oxidative damage

- Anti-parasitic – kills and expels parasitic worms from the intestines

- Anti-rheumatic – helps prevent and relieve arthritis and rheumatism

- Antiseptic – destroys and prevents the growth of microbes

- Anti-spasmodic – relieves smooth muscle spasms

- Anti-viral—inhibits the growth of a virus

- Aphrodisiac – increases or stimulates sexual desire

- Aromatic – has a strong aroma with a high volatile oil content

- Astringent – has a tightening or contracting effect on tissue and a drying effect on mucus secretions

- Carminative – removes gas and bloating from digestive tract and relieves intestinal pain

- Cephalic – remedy for disorders of the head

- Cholagogue – stimulates gallbladder contraction

- Cicatrisant – promotes healing through the formation of scar tissue

- Cordial – stimulant and warming tonic

- Decongestant – reduces nasal mucus production and nasal swelling

- Deodorant – reduces or masks unwanted odors

- Depurative – detoxifying by combatting impurity in the blood and organs

- Diaphoretic – promotes perspiration, reducing fever and helping to eliminate waste through the skin

- Digestive – promotes or aids digestion of food

- Diuretic – increases the production or elimination of urine

- Emmenagogue – stimulates menstrual flow or activity

- Expectorant – soothes bronchial spasm, loosens mucus secretions and helps in their elimination through productive coughing

- Febrifuge – relieves or reduces fever

- Hepatic – aids liver function

- Hormone modulator – balances hormones

- Hypertensive – causes a rise in blood pressure

- Hypotensive – lowers abnormally high blood pressure

- Immune stimulant – stimulates some aspect of the immune system

- Insecticidal – used to repel or kill insects

- Laxative – stimulates bowel movements either by increasing the flow of bile or by stimulating the peristaltic activity of the colon

- Nervine – supports the function of the nervous system

- Restorative – helps to strengthen and revive the body systems

- Rubefacient – increases blood flow when applied to the skin, promoting healing and relieving pain

- Sedative – reduces the functional activity of the nervous system, calming, relaxing

- Stimulant – accelerates the physiological functions and responses of the body

- Styptic – strongly astringent agent that stops or reduces bleeding

- Stomachic – digestive tonic and appetite stimulant

- Sudorific – causes sweating when taken hot and acts like a tonic when taken cold

- Tonic – strengthens and revitalizes

- Uterine tonic – strengthens and revitalizes the uterus and female sexual organs

- Vasoconstrictor – causes narrowing and tightening of blood vessels

- Vasodilator – dilates and relaxes the blood vessels

- Vermifuge – expels parasites from the intestine

- Vulnerary – promotes wound healing and normalizes damaged tissue

Shop at **Mountain Rose Herbs** (www.mountainroseherbs.com) for carrier oils, herbs, clays, salts, containers, and essential oils. Mountain Rose carries books to help you advance your knowledge of essential oils, too.

Don't forget **Amazon** for containers and all ingredients including essential oils. Amazon carries books to help you advance your knowledge of essential oils as well.

Tropical Traditions (www.tropicaltraditions.com) offers good value for coconut oil, carrier oils, and essential oils. A few books on essential oils are included in their limited inventory.

This is not an exhaustive list.

CONTINUING EDUCATION:

For more information on essential oils check out these informative websites:

My website:

<u>**Joybilee Farm**</u> – http://joybileefarm.com

Pop-over to the **Joybilee Farm website** (*http://joybileefarm.com/beginners-guide-to-eo/*) and grab the bonuses including printable botanical posters, a glossary of essential oil actions, discounts, and more essential oil recipes to expand your knowledge and increase your fun, while you learn about your first 10 essential oils.

Education:

Herbal Academy of New England

Blogs:

104 Homestead
Homespun Seasonal Living
Joybilee Farm
Learning and Yearning
Livin' Lovin' Farm
Timber Creek Farm

REFERENCES

Leslie M. Alexander and Linda A. Straub-Bruce. *Dental Herbalism, natural therapies for the mouth*. Healing Arts Press: Rochester, NY, 2014.

Philip Fritchey. *Practical Herbalism, ordinary plants with extraordinary powers*. Whitman Publications: Warsaw, IN, 2004.

Rosemary Gladstar. *Rosemary Gladstar's Herbal Recipes for Vibrant Health, 175 teas, tonics, salves, tinctures, and other natural remedies for the entire family*. Storey Publishing: North Adams, MA, 2008.

Kurt Schnaubelt. *Advanced Aromatherapy, the science of essential oil therapy*. Healing Arts Press: Rochester, NY,1998.

Valerie Ann Wormwood. *The Complete Book of Essential Oils and Aromatherapy, over 600 natural, nontoxic, and fragrant recipes to create health, beauty, and a safe home environment*. New World Library: Novato, CA. 1991.

ABOUT THE AUTHOR:

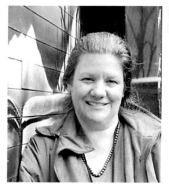

Chris Dalziel is a veteran homeschool Mom with 3 graduates and a published writer, with 30+ years of homesteading under her nails. Living in a log house, in the mountains and surrounded by pines, and pasture, Chris was a city mouse who migrated to the country, as a young mom. Chris is also an award winning fiber-artist who raises her own medium from her organic garden, and from her own sheep. Her passion is to revive the skills and knowledge of the "Lost Arts" of homesteading and self-sufficiency, and present them plainly, so that others can master them and live joyfully, confidently, and courageously in these perilous times.

Herbs and essential oils fascinate Chris. She has been experimenting with essential oils and herbal remedies since she made her first batch of lavender soap in 1982. Her repertoire of essential oil remedies includes blends for pain relief, headache, sinus relief, and digestive aids, as well as DiY cosmetics, healing balms, and natural remedies. To feed her fascination Chris recently completed the **Intermediate Herbal Course** with the **Herbal Academy of New England**. Chris shares her knowledge with her readers on her blog at **JoybileeFarm.com**

Joybilee Farm has been online since 2004. Chris started blogging in 2007. In 2014 the Joybilee Farm blog had 280,000 unique visitors.

Pop-over to the **Joybilee Farm blog**
(*http://joybileefarm.com/beginners-guide-to-eo/*) and grab the bonuses including printable botanical posters, a glossary of essential oil actions, discounts, and more essential oil recipes to give you *confidence in using your first 10 essential oils.*

ACKNOWLEDGEMENTS:

No one writes a book by themselves. This book is the result of much encouragement and mentoring in both book writing and herbal practice. Sarah, I couldn't have finished this project without your encouragement and mentoring. After 21 years of mentoring you, as your homeschool teacher, now the shoe's on the other foot and you are teaching me. I'm indebted to you for proof-reading the manuscript and for your formatting advice in the finished copy, as well as your encouragement to keep going. Your help with making dinner occasionally and baking chocolate chip cookies to fuel the creative process was a tremendous help, too.

There is a group of 4 women that are my constant cheering section, as I go forward in feeling-out this thing that I was made for – writing and learning how to do it better and with intention. Kathie, Angi, Jess, and Tessa this book wouldn't exist if you had not been there to encourage me to keep writing "the book," after all those false starts. Thanks for your writing encouragement and your kind critical eyes in the final drafts. This book is just one tiny part of all that I've written, experimented with, and dreamed of because of your good influence and friendship. Maybe one day we'll all achieve our dreams of seeing our husbands working successfully from home.

Thank you to the Herbal Academy of New England, Amber Meyers – Marketing and Communications Director at HANES, Marlene Adelmann – Director and Founder, Clinical Herbalist & Educator at HANES, and the team at HANES for being interested in my herbal education and in my personal development as a writer and an herbalist. This book is, in part, because of your encouragement and much of the information here was prompted by my studies in the **Intermediate Herbal Course** at HANES.

Angela England, you approached me 2 years ago to write a book on raising Angora rabbits, that I started but never finished. Then you invited me to join you in an online course on writing a book. The Herbal Remedy book I started writing

---

in the course, is still in progress, since it ended up being way longer than I planned. This book was birthed in the middle of that other one. Thanks for being there as a sounding board and as an encourager through the aborted attempts and the final birthing. You are the doula for book birthings. I couldn't have completed this one if you hadn't helped me work through so many others. Thanks for leading the way.

And finally, thank you, reader, for picking up this short book, *The Beginner's Guide to Essential Oils*. I'm so glad to be a part of your journey of learning how to use these amazing natural healing agents in your own home and family. Your energy and enthusiasm for learning all you can is what makes every investment of time and resources in this book worthwhile. Thanks for inviting me along on your personal journey.

If you enjoyed this book, can you please take a few minutes and leave a review on Amazon. I prize your opinion of this work.

Chris Dalziel
Greenwood, BC, Canada

54779153R00075

Made in the USA
San Bernardino, CA
23 October 2017